The Reliable EKG/ECG Interpretation Bible:

Complete & Unique Guide on How to Reliably Carry Out EKG/ECG Interpretation Fast in Few Minutes Even if You are a Novice (Beginner's Guide)

By

Doctor Alex Richmond

Copyright@2018

TABLE OF CONTENT

CHAPTER ONE **3**

INTRODUCTION...3

CHAPTER TWO **8**

THE FUNDAMENTAL ANATOMY OF THE HUMAN

HEART...**8**

CHAPTER THREE **19**

THE BASIC HEART FUNCTION AND THE ECG

PROCESS..19

CHAPTER FOUR **28**

THE BASIC THINGS THAT TRANSPIRE DURING

THE PROCESS OF CARRYING OUT AN ECG 28

CHAPTER FIVE **34**

THE ESSENCE OF HAVING AN ECG, AND ITS

INTERPRETATION 34

THE END

CHAPTER ONE

INTRODUCTION

Meaning of ECG/EKG: This means electrocardiogram, and it is a diagnostic device which is regularly used to get an access to the muscular and electrical functions of the human heart. And the EKG/ECG test is easy to carry out, but needs substantial amount of time in trying to learn it.

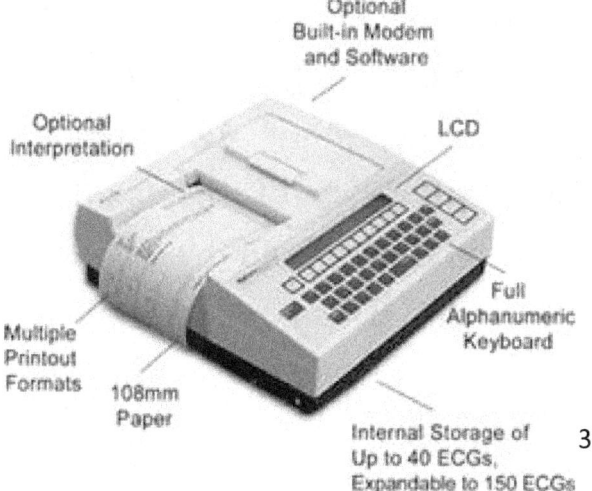

Optional
Built-in Modem
and Software

Optional
Interpretation

LCD

Full
Alphanumeric
Keyboard

Multiple
Printout
Formats

108mm
Paper

Internal Storage of
Up to 40 ECGs,
Expandable to 150 ECGs

Medical studies reveal that the human heart is a two part electrical pump, whose activities could be measured and monitored by simply placing certain electrodes on the skin of the human body. Besides, the rhythm of the human heartbeat, its rate, together with the flow of flow of blood to the heart muscle can all be measured.

An approved method has been created when it comes to carrying out a regular EKG/ ECG. Importantly, the 12 unique electrical views of the human heart are produced by just 10 electrodes which are placed at certain parts of the body. On each leg and arm a single electrode lead is placed there. And of course on the wall of the chest six electrode leads are there. Also, the unique signals that emanate from each of the electrode lead are immediately recorded by the device. And on the electrocardiogram you we see the printed views of the recordings which are shown on the device.

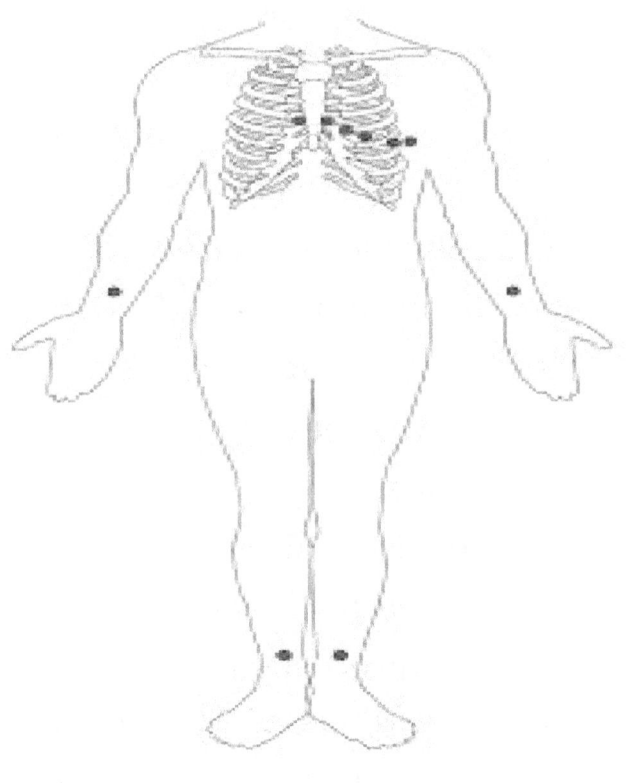

In contrast, monitoring a human heart needs just 3 leads; with one each on the left chest, right arm and the left arm. Besides, this does not make up a complete ECG since it only carries out the measurement of rhythm and rate of the heart.

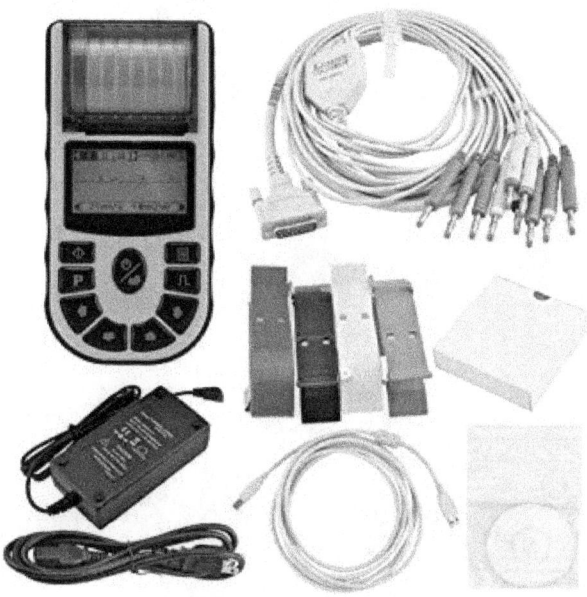

CHAPTER TWO
THE FUNDAMENTAL ANATOMY OF THE HUMAN HEART

Human Heart

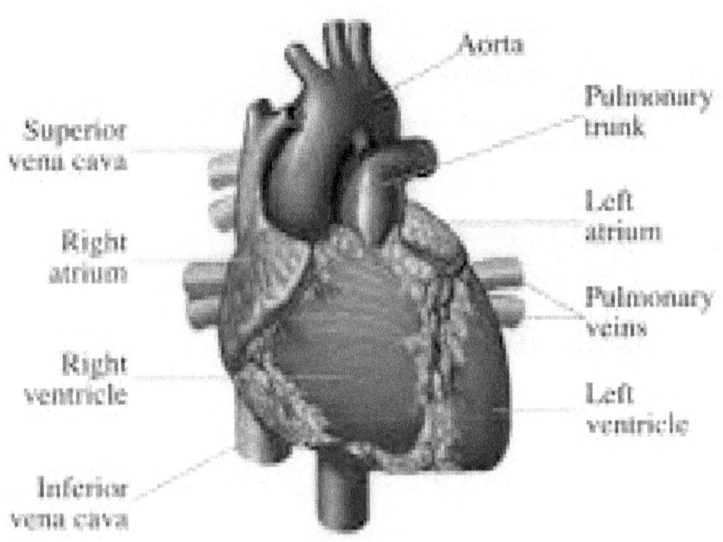

Superior vena cava

Right atrium

Right ventricle

Inferior vena cava

Aorta

Pulmonary trunk

Left atrium

Pulmonary veins

Left ventricle

Interestingly, the human heart consists of four special chambers, which include: the left and the right ventricles, and the left atrium and right atrium. In addition, the right part of the human heart takes blood from the body and quickly gives it to the lungs whereas, the left part of the human heart collects blood from the lungs and eventually gives this to the human body.

Importantly, the flow of blood through the entire body goes thus:

*Blood rich in oxygen which comes from the lungs goes into the left atrium via the pulmonary veins of the heart.

*This blood then goes into the left ventricle where the blood is further given to the aorta, and it is thereafter taken to other parts of the body.
*The de-oxygenated blood returns to the human heart, it comes with carbon dioxide which is a waste product of the metabolic process. This blood comes in through the right atrium, where the blood is received and given to the right ventricle of the heart

*Finally, the right ventricle of the heart then passes the blood via the pulmonary artery to the lungs where the compound, carbon dioxide, is removed and oxygen is immediately replaced and the process or cycle goes on and on.

Similar to every other muscle, the human heart needs nutrients and oxygen to carry out its function effectively. Consequently, nutrient and oxygen are supplied via the arteries that come from the aorta, which is also found in the heart. More so, the blood vessels go out to deliver to all the parts of heart the oxygenated blood.

From the electrical dimension, the human heart is sectioned into two, namely the lower chamber or section and the upper chamber or section. The signal created in the upper section of the human heart brings about the atria squeezing and bringing the blood into the ventricles of the heart. The ventricles are filled up with the help of a short delay, thereafter; the ventricles immediately come together and pump blood to the lung and the other parts of the body for normal activities.

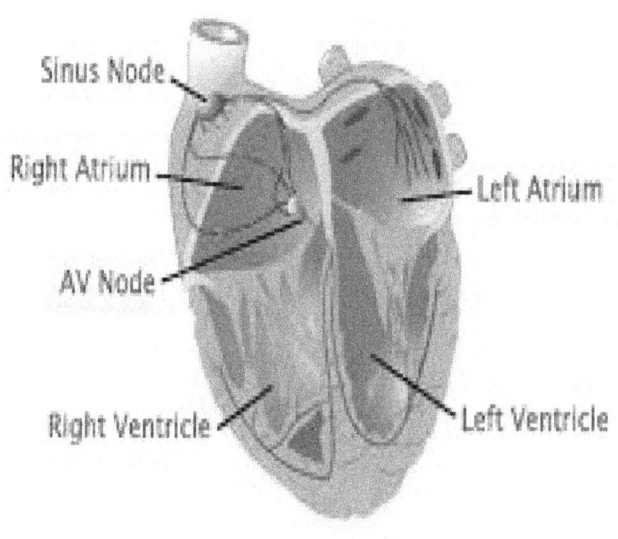

Note the following salient acronyms which will be used in the course of our explanations:

*LB means left bundle

*RB means right bundle

*SA means sinoatrial node

*AV means atrioventricular node

Carrying out system conduction of the human heart-

The LB and RB are the nerves that carry the electrical impulse or signals from AV nodes straight to the ventricles of the human heart.

The SA node which is located in the right part of the atrium, works without depending on the brain to create electricity for the human heart to work effectively or to beat accordingly.

Note the following activities or electrical signals that are generated in the human heart:

*Originally, the signals created by the SA node goes through the electrical grid of the heart and gives signals to the muscle cells found in the atria, to beat at the same time, and this gives room for a sequential squeeze of the human heart during the process. And as the atria contrast, it forces blood into the ventricles of the human heart.

*More so, the signals created in the SA node move to a point between the ventricles and the atria where is slowed down for few milliseconds to give the ventricles time to fill up.

*These signals then move through the ventricle of the heart, and this brings a kind of stimulation that results in the contraction of the muscle cells of the human heart. And this contraction of the ventricle takes blood to the lungs, from the right part of the ventricle, and to the human body, from the left part of the ventricle.

*Finally, a short pause seems to take place to allow blood to go back to the human heart and occupy it before a repetition of the entire process or cycle. And this will immediately take you to

the next expected hear beat.
That is it!

CHAPTER THREE

THE BASIC HEART FUNCTION AND THE ECG PROCESS

Essentially, the leads of electrode placed on the wall of the human chest are able to carry out a detection of the electrical signals or impulses created by the human heart. And the electrical and clear views of the human heart are provided by the multiple leads. And through the interpretation of the trace, a doctor understands the heart rhythm and its rate together with the flow of blood to the ventricle of the heart.

Explanation of Rhythm and Rate

The heart rhythm simply has to do with kind of heart beat. And the human heart beat in a rhythm referred to as a sinus rhythm, and in which each electrical signal created by the SA leads to a heart beat or contrast in the ventricle. Importantly, when we have series of electrical rhythm that are not normal; some could be very dangerous while others are okay. More so, certain electrical rhythms will not create a heartbeat. Therefore they are very terrible and are majorly responsible for sudden death that happens around us.

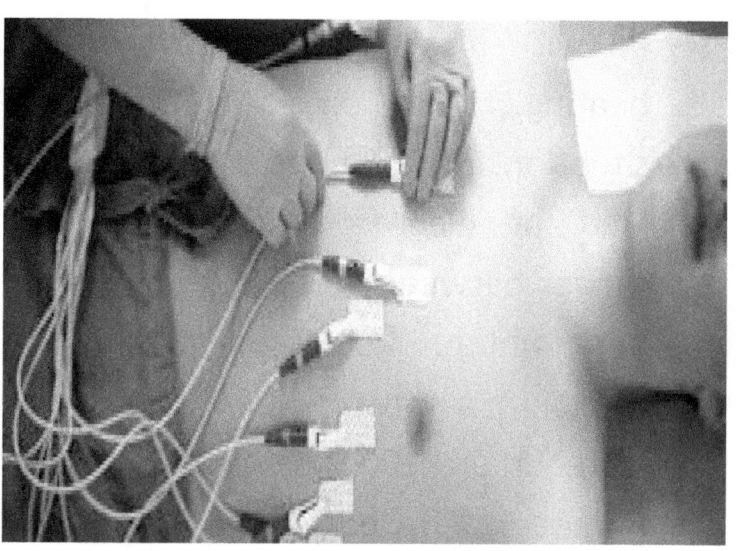

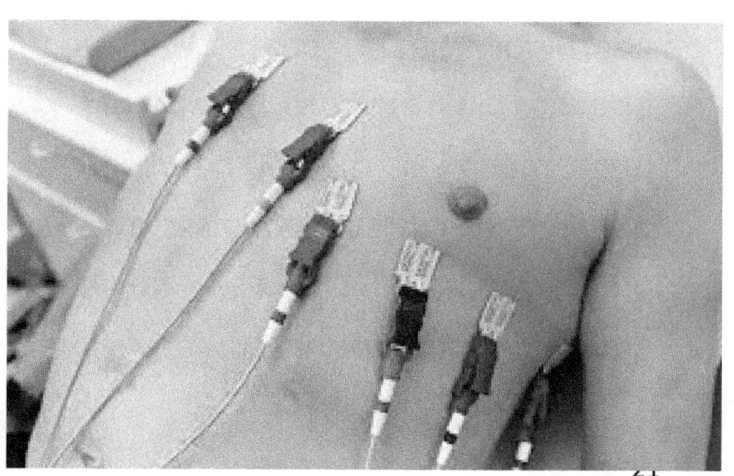

In addition, the heart rate has to do with how fast the heart is beating. And on a normal situation, the SA node creates a kind of electrical signal that ranges between 50 to 100 times per minute. Also, Tachycardia refers to a rate of heart much faster than 100 beats in one minute; tachy equals fast plus cardia which is now equal to heart or heart beat. While bradycardia refers to a rate of heart much less than 50 beats in one minute; brady equals slow plus cardia which also now equals the heart or heartbeat.

The heart rhythm examples include the following:

*Sinus tachycardia

*Normal sinus rhythm

*sinus bradycardia

*Atrial flutter

*Atrial fibrillation

*Ventricular tachycardia

*Ventricular fibrillation

More so, with regard to the transmission of electrical signal or impulse to any place in the system, delays are usually involved. And certain signal or impulse leads to the heart rhythm where you have normal or usual variants, and others could threaten one's life, e.g

*Left bundle branch block

*Right bundle branch block

*First degree AV block

*Second degree AV block (type 2)

*Second degree AV block (type 1, Wenckebach)

*Complete heart block or third degree AV block

ST segment

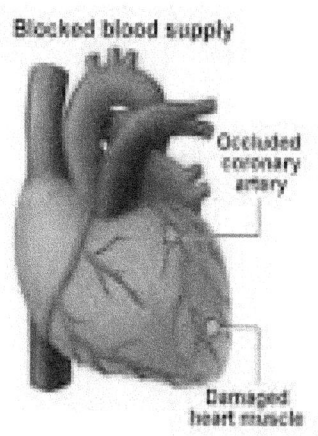

Blocked blood supply

Occluded coronary artery

Damaged heart muscle

- ST changes from baseline can indicate bad things for the heart
- ST depression indicates ischemia
- ST elevation indicates injury or infarct
- *Also beware the sloping ST segment*

Additionally, there could be cases of short circuits that can result to abnormal electrical signals in the human heart, which can further results in rhythm and rate abnormalities.

The WPW, *Wolfe Parkinson White*, syndrome is a medical situation in which an abnormality in the pathway of node of AV can lead to a situation called tachycardia, which was earlier mentioned above.

Importantly, the trace from ECG can give us relevant information like knowing whether the muscle cells of the human heart are conducting electricity accordingly. And through the analysis of the waves of electrical signal, your doctor is able to know if there a decrease in the flow of blood to vital areas likes the muscles of the human heart. Besides, heart attack or myocardial is related to acute or serious blockages, which can also be determined in the process as well. Consequently, when someone presents the issue of chest pain to a doctor or physician an ECG test is immediately done to find out what is actually happening.

CHAPTER FOUR

THE BASIC THINGS THAT TRANSPIRE DURING THE PROCESS OF CARRYING OUT AN ECG

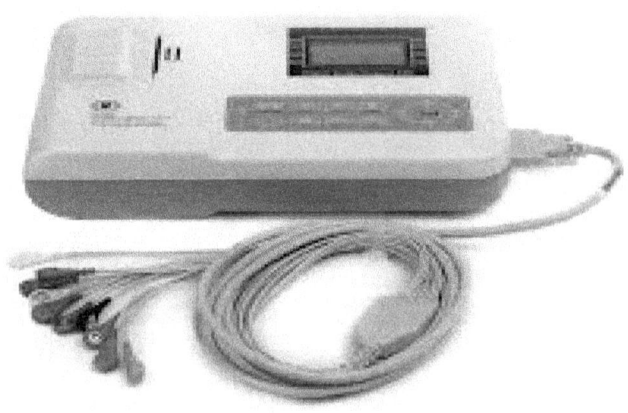

As we have said before now, the ECG is easy to carry out but you need to master the intricacies involved it; it will not harm you and it is not invasive. In carry out the test, certain patches are quickly placed on the patient's skin to immediately carry out the detection of electrical signs or impulse that is generated in the human heart. And an ECG device or machine simultaneously carries out the recording of these electrical signs or impulses that are generated. As we have also explained before now a patch is placed on each leg and one also on each shoulder. That is to say, the limbs of the patient have four patches placed on them; such patches or leads are called the limb leads. On the wall of the chest six patches are place here during the process, starting with the right part of the breast bone, and of course they are referred to as chest leads since they are placed on the chest. On an ECG device or machine, the patches mentioned above are connected to the machine which does the recording of these traces. And after the entire process, the traces are eventually printed on paper to show the results of the test.

Interestingly, modern ECG machines or devices now have special video screen that assists health personnel in ascertaining whether the traces are sufficient enough or to ascertain whether such tests should under repetition.

Although, they may not completely be a perfect one, but are now incorporated with computer programs that assist in the interpretation of the ECG tests.

In carry out the test, the patient's skin should be dry and neat to prevent the interference of the electrical signals, and to have traces that can be accepted for one's interpretation given out by the machine.

Things to avoid or carry out

It should be noted that in carrying out the process, one may be required to aggressively clean skin with a towel or you may be required to shave chest hair depending on the situation. And it should also be noted that the equality of ECG traces may also be affected by interference which can be caused by tremors or shivering. So patients should try as much as possible to avoid this or should be told about the interference.   Consequently, patients are told to be still and steady for 5 to 10 seconds without movement in order to get the needed and appropriate results for the ECG tests.

CHAPTER FIVE

THE ESSENCE OF HAVING AN ECG, AND ITS INTERPRETATION

Normal vs Abnormal ECG

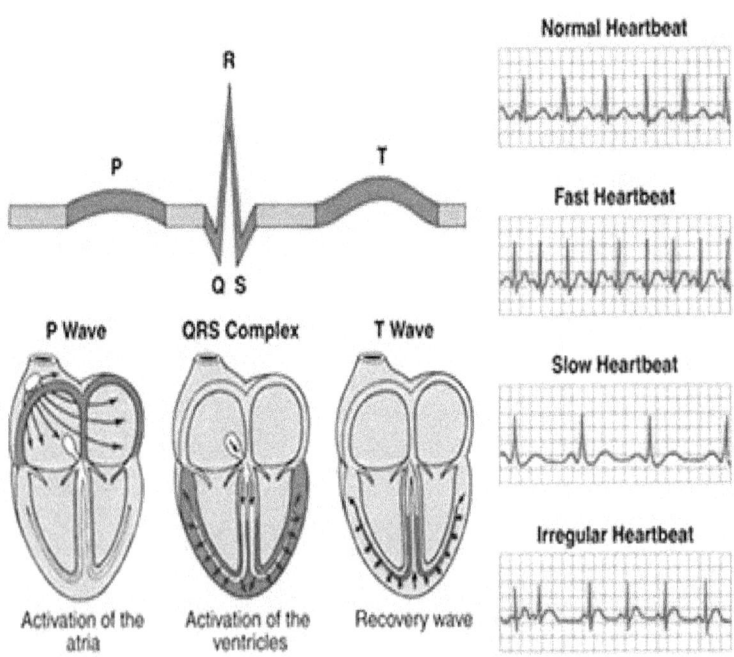

The Essence of an ECG Test

As we have mentioned before now, the function of the human heart is accessed with the help or assistance of an ECG or ECG test. And it is used to assess patient's shortness of breath or chest pains; such test will reveal if the patients are having or are likely to have heart attack or acute myocardial infarction.

The ECG test may assist in deciding whether a particular pain is a medical condition called angina or as a result of narrowing of the patient's blood vessels leading to the patient's heart. Besides, in trying to find out an abnormality, a series of EKG tests may be required over time; this will facilitate getting accurate results.

In addition, since abnormality of the heart rhythm and heart rate is capable of affecting the capability of the human heart to give out blood and render the body the oxygen that it needs to function it is important to note that when a patient is complaining about things like passing out (syncope), light-headedness, and palpitations, ECG tests should immediately be conducted on such a patient to ascertain the cause of these signs.

The Interpretation of an ECG

Here, this demands for a good level of experience and education. In diagnosing a heart ailment or disease, physical examination and history are very relevant in doing this. If ECG is normal or usual, physician discussion with the patient in question will be of great importance as it will reveal the possibility of a heart issues or problems. Also, the ECG tests or assessments are as follows:

*Assessing the rhythm of the heart.

*Finding out how the electrical patterns of conduction look like; the conduction of electrical signals by a normal heart muscle is quite different from an abnormal one. Since the abnormal conduction is seen during the recovery of the ventricles and the contraction of the ventricles.

*Determining the heart rate.

Furthermore, the human heart tracing or traces in twelve lead is recorded by the ECG machine. That is, six chest leads of V1 to

V6 and also six limb leads of Iii, II, I, AVF, AVR and AVL.

It should be noted the P wave concentrates on atria. And T wave solves the recovery of ventricular stage as they are re-occupied with blood. And as for the QRS complex concentrates on the ventricles.

It is should be noted that the PR interval assists in the measurement of the time it takes for electrical signals to move from the SA node to the AV node during the time of the test. The QT interval assists in the measurement of how long it will take the ventricles to undergo recovery, and get ready for the next beat. And for QRS interval, it measures the time of electrical move or travel via the ventricles.

The fundamental P-QRS-T wave pattern or sequence: Here, the strip reveals a sequence in which 1 square equals 0.04 sec/0.1mV. This is shown below.

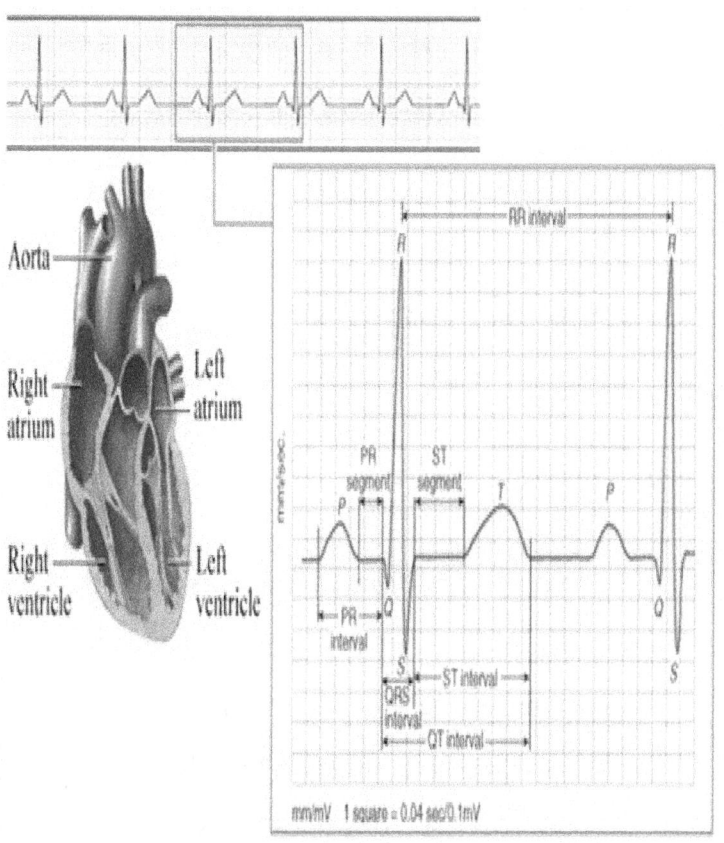

The measurement of the time it takes for the electrical signals to move from the node of the SA to the ventricles is carried out by a computer which is incorporated in the ECG device or machine.

And measurements like these greatly assist physicians in knowing certain kinds of heart block and also assist the physician in assessing the heart rate.

In the interpretation process, artificial intelligence or computer programs can be of immense help as their results are most times accurate. On the other hand, the human factor is still of high relevance as it help in the assessment process.

As regards decision making when it comes to ECG results, it

depends both on the ECG traces or tracing and clinical condition. And on a normal ground, the ECG will not exclude disease of the heart, and for the ECG that is abnormal may perhaps be the *normal baseline* for such persons.

Some Other Relevant ECG Diagrams

They are given below:

*The *12 lead* ECG of a patient with pain in chest. This reveals acute inferior wall myocardial infarction or heart attack as shown below.

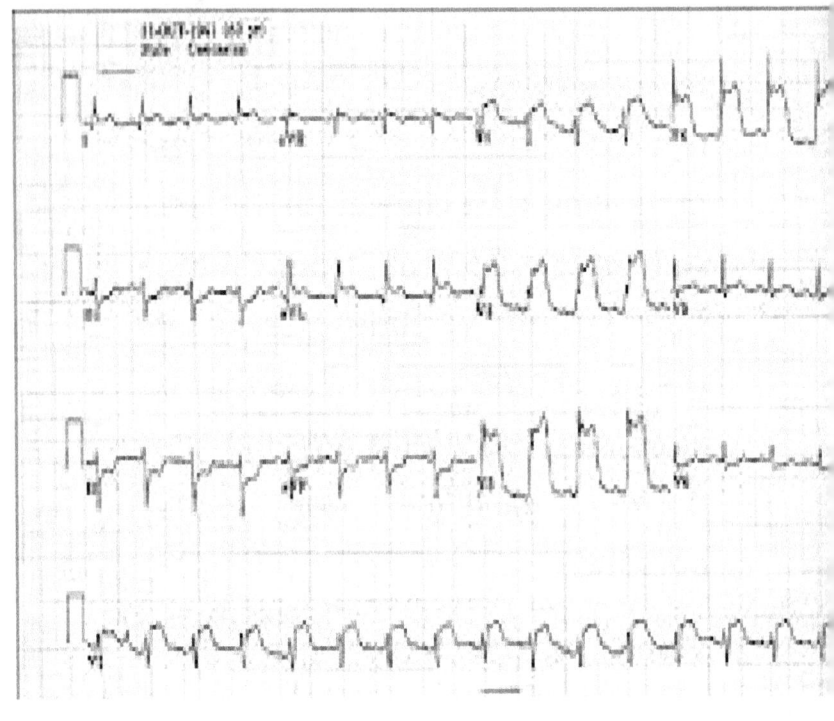

*The rhythm stripes of a patient that was cardioverted by a strong electric shock is shown below.

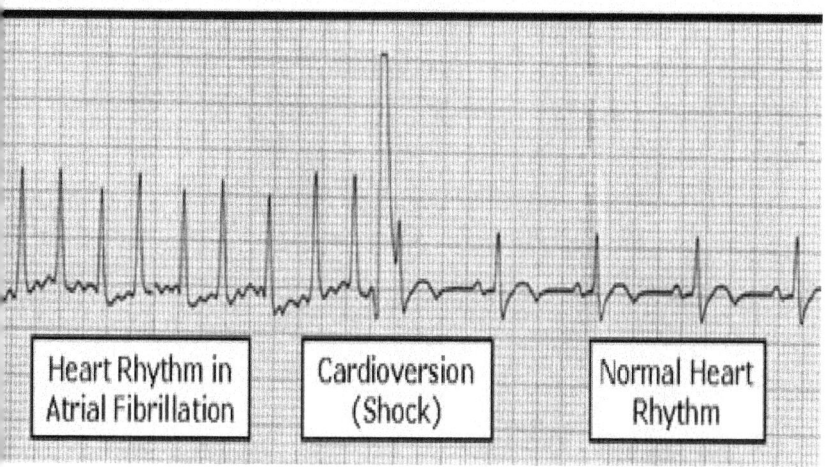

Heart Rhythm in Atrial Fibrillation | Cardioversion (Shock) | Normal Heart Rhythm

Other books written by the same authors:

1) www.amazon.com/dp/B078L4LBKS

2) www.amazon.com/dp/1982007753

3) www.amazon.com/dp/1982040858

4) www.amazon.com/dp/1981863400

5) www.amazon.com/dp/1983462918

6) www.amazon.com/dp/1983496332

7) www.amazon.com/dp/B079QYRV5R

8)www.amazon.com/dp/B07C2QNK9C

9) www.amazon.com/dp/B07C63PVLV

10) www.amazon.com/dp/B07C2QNK9C

THE END

CPSIA information can be obtained
at www.ICGtesting.com
Printed in the USA
BVHW04s0743240618
519880BV00006B/470/P